LEARN EVERYTHING YOU NEED TO LOSE FAT AND GAIN MUSCLE AT THE SAME TIME

EVEN AS A COMPLETE BEGINNER, WITH THE SEVEN KEYS TO STRENGTH TRAINING FOR MEN OVER 50

BRYANT WILLIS

Contents

Chapter 1

THE BEGINNING OF A JOURNEY

Everyone ages. Aging is unavoidable and will affect everyone at some point. Some people may handle this process gracefully, while others may want to hang onto their youth as long as they can. It is an unavoidable reality of the world in which we live. Additionally, there are a number of effects of aging that we must manage, including:

Each day, more and more of our muscular mass is lost.

Our bones weaken with time.

The normal decrease of testosterone that occurs in the body affects many other things.

I am a great believer in self-acceptance and being proud of who you are, but that doesn't mean you have to give in to your circumstances. We construct our own pathways through life, and becoming older won't be able to stop us. The ability to exert effort is all that is necessary to overcome these natural laws. You may retaliate and regain control of your life with my assistance.

In her 30s, Clara was a buddy of mine from long ago. She had recently wed James, a widower with two children from his deceased wife who was in his early 50s. When James and Clara first met, it was love at first sight at one of my friend's parties. Despite having a gap of more than 15 years, you could see they were truly connected. It was clear. They started dating and made the decision to intensify their relationship by getting married. James claimed he wasn't "in the mood" when they first started having issues in the bedroom before they got married. She waited for him in the hopes that this phase will pass because my friend Clara is a charming and patient person. They were married for a few months without any problems. Clara, who had been mistreated by her ex, started thinking about meeting him again out of desperation, and not just for sex. James was unable to sate her sexually. He hadn't liked what he saw when he looked in the mirror. He was intensely aware of the age difference and its consequences on his body in bed, and he felt inadequate. Although Clara did not feel this way, James believed it made him less appealing to her. Despite the fact that James already deeply believed this, Clara did not feel this way.

A deadly misunderstanding occurred because Clara believed he had lost interest in her. She looked to her ex, Dan, once more for what she couldn't find in James. One day, as we were chatting, she confided in me about her predicament. I had a clear understanding of the situation, so I said, "A simple problem to solve." I pleaded with her to let me step in. James and I became friends, and I asked him to some of my workouts and enrolled him in consistent training. Over time, James's perspective changed; he gained the self-assurance to face himself in the mirror and be proud of the person he saw. His lover and he enjoyed a wonderful sexual relationship as a result of his confidence. They were no longer in control of his life, therefore he was able to voice to Clara his past worries about his physique. Their bond is greater than ever right now.

I feel a wide range of feelings as I think back on this incident. Even though everything turned out okay in the end, their marriage might have ended because of that issue. James had low testosterone levels, which adversely affected his sexual desire and his capacity to engage in enjoyable sex. This was completely unknown to him. Because it improves muscle mass, regular exercise can increase testosterone levels. More testosterone may be produced by the body when muscle mass increases. It is my goal to get you there since strength training becomes increasingly important as you age due to various factors, including testosterone.

James is one of many men who, like James, struggle with aging-related muscle loss, fat accumulation, and strength loss, making it difficult for them to carry out their everyday duties. When your lack of fitness prohibits you from performing tasks that you once did with ease, it can be very irritating. Unfortunately, some people believe they are too old to start exercising and that their age prevents them from building muscle or shedding fat. In actuality, you must maintain your fitness regardless of your age, and I'd even venture to suggest that it becomes even more crucial as you get older.

You are not past your prime for a workout. No of your age, maintaining a healthy weight is essential for both your physical and mental wellbeing. Your ability to manage daily tasks grows more difficult as you age, and it gets worse if you don't lead a fit lifestyle. There are several myths about the kinds of fitness activities that persons between the ages of 50 and 70 can engage in. Because of how our bodies are built, as we age, fitness may not be as heavily focused on extensive training sessions to carve off the abs. Instead, the exercises I teach are geared on keeping you in shape and reducing your risk of developing cardiovascular problems. while also enhancing your balance and muscle mass. It is crucial to be aware of your health, strength, and fitness as you reach the age of 50 and beyond.

Lack of exercise or a lack of commitment to exercise can lead to a variety of health problems. As we age, these problems grow increasingly challenging. Lack of exercise can cause muscles to stiffen, which can cause pain and discomfort when moving. Having said that, I don't want you to feel discouraged or despair over your age, lack of exercise, or irregular exercise routine after reading all of this. There is always time. Even as a young man, you can achieve a healthy, athletic lifestyle and have that amazing figure you always wanted!

I need you to do me a favor right now. Please decide consciously to act on this book's advice and give yourself the resolve to lead a healthy lifestyle. Worry less about the likelihood of getting hurt because this book's knowledge will give you all you need to train as safely as possible and put an end to injuries. The majority of the drive you require is included in this book, but the remaining portion must come from you. If you take my advise and read through each chapter, you should be well on your way to developing into the physically strong and healthy man that everyone admires. Thankfully, you don't have to do it by yourself. This book will walk you through the seven essential steps to getting the body of your dreams. I'm sure you'll have gathered a ton of knowledge you can use in your life by the time this book is up, and I'll have won your trust.

By purchasing this book, you have chosen well if you are new to fitness and strength training. Just over ten years ago, I started working as an instructor in the fitness industry. My desire is to support you in achieving all of your physical objectives. To be clear, it doesn't have to be difficult or require spending a lot of time in the gym; all you need is the willpower to persevere through the difficult parts. I put together this book because I want to assist you in doing it correctly. I have acquired information about fitness in general and, specifically, men's fitness between the ages of 40 and above via years of experience. I am aware of the enormous advantages of exercising your body and making positive changes in your life.

Okay, so now that you are familiar with me and what I have to offer, I hope you can appreciate the importance of this book. So let's get started without further ado!

Chapter 2

5 O U N D E R S T A N D I N G THE P O W E R O F S T R E N G T H T R A I N I N N G

You could hurt yourself if you believe that starting is useless because you missed your chance. Wrong. Opportunities will always knock on your door. It's never too late to start a practice, alter or improve a bad attitude, launch a business or career, and many other things.

Does Dwight Muhammad Qawi know you? Dwight had a fantastic career at the top of the heap despite beginning his profession at a young age in terms of boxing. At the incredibly late age of 25, Dwight eventually started participating in the sport. Even worse, he began his adventure while incarcerated in Rahway State Prison for armed robbery. As you would imagine, this man's life had reached its lowest point. The majority of individuals wouldn't anticipate him to ever achieve anything. But no matter what, there is always a path out of the shadows. He emerged from the pit of despair and went on to win world championships in the light-heavyweight and cruiserweight weight classifications. Tim Thomas, Randy Johnson, Didier Drogba, Antonio Gates, Bill Durnan, Hakeem Olajuwon, and Kurt Warner are just a few examples of sportsmen that entered their respective sports later than others but still managed to leave their impact on history. There are tens of thousands more.

Strength training definition

Strength training, as I would define it, is any physical activity intended to enhance muscular growth or fitness in a particular muscle area. It is an exercise that stresses the engaged muscles by applying a resistance force.

It entails giving your muscles more attention than they often receive. Your muscles are overworked. Any activity that targets the body's major muscular groups with a medium to high level of effort qualifies as strength training. You should be aware that strength training involves more than just using weights in a gym to bulk up. Much more is involved than that.

Older strength athletes can be broken down into three groups: those who never quit working out, those who relapsed, and those who never worked out at all. But as you become older—more over 50—strength training has indisputable advantages. Everybody can benefit from strength training, especially those with health conditions including obesity, high or low blood sugar levels, heart disease, arthritis, and many others. Strength training is an important component of the body's total fitness. Studies have demonstrated that strength training can help older adults who are physically feeble and have weak muscles.

Strength Training Methods

Strength training comes in a variety of forms, including isometric, isotonic, and isokinetic exercises. If you're still unclear as to what any of this means, don't worry. Let me clarify.

Exercises for Isometric Strength: Additionally called static strength training. Without actually extending or shortening the muscles, this sort of exercise recruits muscles and exerts stress. Your muscles are flexed, but they are not contracting or expanding. Exercises for isometric training frequently target your entire body. Additionally, it's appropriate to engage your complete body simultaneously in tasks. If you need a variation from your usual fitness regimen or have trouble with your knees, isometric exercises are a great option. Plank and side bridge, wall sit, and other yoga postures including the chair and tree poses are all examples of isometric exercise. However, because these exercises increase strength in a single body position, they should be used in conjunction with more dynamic training programs.

Strength training that is isotonic maintains the muscle's tension or tone even as it is shortened You may think of a lot of isotonic exercises. You are purposefully extending your body across a range of motion while resisting an external weight or force. The majority of the isotonic exercise routine, including squats, pull-ups, push-ups, stair climbing, deadlifts, etc., are probably familiar to you.

Isokinetic Strength Training: This type of exercise forces you to move through a range of motion continuously. The majority of isokinetic exercise is performed on specialized machines that generate a constant force regardless of the amount of effort you put out. The equipment regulates the exercise's tempo by varying resistance over the course of your predetermined range of motion. No matter how hard you try, your speed or mobility doesn't change. You can tune the speed and range of motion to a target that best suits your requirements. Your muscular strength and endurance can be tested and enhanced through isokinetic training. Isokinetic exercise is best exemplified by using a stationary bike, which you may obtain at your neighborhood gym.

Testosterone as a Factor

Most men over 50 seem to lose their vigor, power, and energy with time. But it shouldn't be the case. The frailty and decreased energy that we frequently associate with aging include challenges with climbing, carrying burdens, and long distance walking. And each of these is mostly brought on by muscle loss. Inactivity is, in fact, one of the primary causes of muscular muscle loss. I'll give you an illustrative example. Pitch two men in their mid-50s, one who has spent years exercising and using his body, the other who spends most of his time watching old movies while seated in front of the television. Consider a situation in which you requested them to carry out a duty that they had never done before but that required some physical effort and flexibility. Who do you think does that task more effectively? The person who has consistently put effort into strength training will do better. With ease, too. You might think that this situation is apparent, but let's explore it further. First off, his body is not unfamiliar with the task and has become accustomed to performing the type of movements; second, his endurance is significantly higher, indicating that his body is well prepared to withstand the effort. This is one instance where the proverb "you either use them or lose them" applies to muscles. Your ability to perform any physical work will improve if you keep your muscles active. And by far, one of the finest methods to build those muscles is through strength training.

As we become older, testosterone levels inevitably decline in all males. A urologist at UW Health's Males's Health Clinic named David Paolone wrote in a paper that about 39% of men over the age of 45 have low testosterone. A low concentration is one that is less than 300 nanograms per deciliter. And low testosterone is more common as men age, affecting 12 percent of men in their 50s, 19 percent in their 60s, 28 percent in their 70s, and 49 percent in their 80s, according to estimates (UW Health, 2017).

Let me clarify testosterone for those who are confused. Both humans and other animals produce this hormone. The essential male sex hormone is it (also found in females but with a much lower concentration). The main source of testosterone in men is the testicles. In addition to regulating sex drive, it is essential for the development of sperm, fertility, muscle mass, bone density, fat distribution, and red blood cells. I believe you can now appreciate the significance of this hormone. During puberty, testosterone production rises, and it begins to decline beyond the age of 30. Men's testosterone levels begin to gradually decline after the age of 30 at a pace of, on average, about 1% every year. Aging naturally causes testosterone levels to decline. There are numerous effects of testosterone. When it falls below a particular level that is regarded as healthy, it might cause hypogonadism (a condition where the body doesn't generate enough male hormones or sperm) or infertility. Loss of muscular mass is a severe side effect of low testosterone.

Reduced hormone levels can cause a considerable loss of muscle because testosterone is crucial for the growth and regulation of muscle mass. Although low testosterone reduces muscular mass, it has no effect on the muscles' ability to work or their strength. Simply put, muscle mass refers to all of your body's muscles, including your skeletal, smooth, and cardiac muscles. There are risks to your health if you have low muscle mass. Your general health may suffer as a result.

Low muscle mass is linked to worse outcomes, including more post-operative and surgical problems, a longer hospital stay, decreased physical function, a lower quality of life, and shorter survival.

2021 — WITHINGS

Strength training's advantages

Many men believe that lifting weights is just useful for developing their biceps and desired six-pack. Maybe that's one of the reasons older men won't think about it. They aren't really concerned with how their body appears or how other people view them. Although I want to emphasize that this lifestyle is totally fine, strength training goes above and beyond. Strength training is crucial if you want to develop bigger biceps. Strength training is still one of the best strategies to achieve your health goals, even if reaching your maximum muscle size isn't your goal. Let me go through some of the advantages of strength training before your next workout so you can approach it and following sessions with an understanding of why you subject your body to it.

Fitness and strength.

Even though this is extremely evident, we cannot ignore it. You become fitter and stronger with strength training. Muscle strength is essential for performing daily duties, especially as you approach your fifties and naturally start to lose muscle mass. Strength training reduces the possibility of experiencing trouble carrying out daily tasks because of a lack of physical fitness. These regular activities could include stair ascending and stair descending, lifting heavy furniture or other objects, participating in sports or trekking, or even just standing still for extended periods of time. Simply said, when you're not fit and unable to perform the activities you enjoy to the best of your ability, it takes the enjoyment out of them.

protection of muscle mass and bone health.

As mentioned previously, we begin to lose an average of 1% of our lean muscle mass every year after we reach the age of 30 or so. In a 2017 study for Bone and Mineral Research, it was discovered that 30 minutes twice a week of high-intensity resistance and impact exercise increased functional performance. Additionally, postmenopausal women with poor bone mass had higher bone density, shape, and strength without experiencing any negative side effects (Watson, Weeks, Weis, Harding, Horan, Beck, 2017). Additionally, the HHS recommendations state that strength training exercises benefit everyone by maintaining or gaining muscle mass, which is important for maintaining bone, joint, and muscle health as we age (U.S. Department of Health and Human Services, 2018).

controls excessive weight

Since strength training is not centered on shedding pounds by burning as many calories as possible, it may put them off since this is a common misconception. There are a lot more types of exercise that put this first. For instance, cardiovascular exercise like running, swimming, or walking increases the amount of calories your body burns; this will definitely help you lose weight. But even if you're not burning as many calories throughout your workouts, strength training is still beneficial. Numerous studies support the idea that strength training aids in weight loss by boosting your resting metabolism. Your excess post-exercise oxygen usage rises after a successful strength training session. After a strength training session, your body keeps burning calories. Strength training keeps your metabolism going considerably longer than aerobic exercise does. In a 2017 study on "Obesity," three groups of dieters were observed: those who did no exercise, those who engaged in only aerobic activity, and those who undertook strength training activities four times per week for 18 months. Strength-training dieters dropped the most fat, on average 18 pounds. Compared to dieters who didn't exercise who only dropped 10 pounds, aerobic exercisers shed 16 pounds!

Development of Better Body Mechanics

Your posture, coordination, and balance all improve. Older persons have lower physical functioning, which increases their risk of falling. Through a strength training exercise, you can significantly lower your chance of falling. Body balance is a function of how well your stabilizing muscles are working. Your balance will be greater and steadier the more muscular you are.

Osteoporosis Management and Prevention

A prevalent medical problem in older persons is osteoporosis.

The disease weakens the bones, increasing the risk of fracture. People frequently are unaware of it because it can take years to develop.

Strong bones are a feature of muscles. Your bone mineral density is considerably increased by strength training. Exercises that involve bearing weight and gravity pressing down on your body put stress on your joints and muscles. Additionally, each time a muscle contracts, it pulls on the bone that is connected to it, causing the bone cell to release structural proteins that transport minerals into the bone. Focus on standing weight-bearing exercises like lunges and squats if you want to achieve remarkable improvements in this area. Just 12 weeks of strength training with squats raised the bone mineral density of the lower spine and femur (thigh) by 2.9 and 4.9 percent, respectively, in a 2014 Journal of Family and Community Medicine study.

Control of Chronic Illnesses

The multiple advantages of strength training to treat different health problems have been well-documented in numerous research. It has been demonstrated that strength training can aid in the management of chronic illnesses. Strength training can be just as beneficial as medication at reducing arthritis pain if you have it. Strength training can help stabilize your blood sugar levels and increase how well your body uses insulin whether you have low or high blood sugar.I'd want to introduce myself before telling you about a brief book I wrote to go along with what you're about to read. A balanced diet is the basis of ultimate fitness. To help you reduce fat and maintain a healthy body, I have created a meal plan.

I did, however, feel that it would be unjust and a little ungrateful to push a sale after you had just purchased one of my books. I've chosen to give you this one for free instead.

Here is a little glimpse of the benefits you will experience from this free book:

A full day's worth of delectable meals prepared for you that are intended to help you lose weight

Various menu options will keep things interesting and prevent boredom.

Important information on which meals to consume and which to avoid in order to become an authority on weight loss

You might as well peek inside because it's free, as I just mentioned. It's a really simple procedure. Simply click the link below to be sent to a page where you can enter your email address, and I'll send it right to you. The website is bryantjwillis.com.

Hope you enjoy it!

T HE B E G I N N I N G O F A JOU R N E Y

Everyone ages. Aging is unavoidable and will affect everyone at some point. Some people may handle this process gracefully, while others may want to hang onto their youth as long as they can. It is an unavoidable reality of the world in which we live. Additionally, there are a number of effects of aging that we must manage, including:

Each day, more and more of our muscular mass is lost.

Our bones weaken with time.

The normal decrease of testosterone that occurs in the body affects many other things.

I am a great believer in self-acceptance and being proud of who you are, but that doesn't mean you have to give in to your circumstances. We construct our own pathways through life, and becoming older won't be able to stop us. The ability to exert effort is all that is necessary to overcome these natural laws. You may retaliate and regain control of your life with my assistance.

In her 30s, Clara was a buddy of mine from long ago. She had recently wed James, a widower with two children from his deceased wife who was in his early 50s. When James and Clara first met, it was love at first sight at one of my friend's parties. Despite having a gap of more than 15 years, you could see they were truly connected. It was clear. They started dating and made the decision to intensify their relationship by getting married. James claimed he wasn't "in the mood" when they first started having issues in the bedroom before they got married. She waited for him in the hopes that this phase will pass because my friend Clara is a charming and patient person. They were married for a few months without any problems. Clara, who had been mistreated by her ex, started thinking about meeting him again out of desperation, and not just for sex. James was unable to sate her sexually. He hadn't liked what he saw when he looked in the mirror. He was intensely aware of the age difference and its consequences on his body in bed, and he felt inadequate. Although Clara did not feel this way, James believed it made him less appealing to her. Despite the fact that James already deeply believed this, Clara did not feel this way.

A deadly misunderstanding occurred because Clara believed he had lost interest in her. She looked to her ex, Dan, once more for what she couldn't find in

James. One day, as we were chatting, she confided in me about her predicament. I had a clear understanding of the situation, so I said, "A simple problem to solve." I pleaded with her to let me step in. James and I became friends, and I asked him to some of my workouts and enrolled him in consistent training. Over time, James's perspective changed; he gained the self-assurance to face himself in the mirror and be proud of the person he saw. His lover and he enjoyed a wonderful sexual relationship as a result of his confidence. They were no longer in control of his life, therefore he was able to voice to Clara his past worries about his physique. Their bond is greater than ever right now.

I feel a wide range of feelings as I think back on this incident. Even though everything turned out okay in the end, their marriage might have ended because of that issue. James had low testosterone levels, which adversely affected his sexual desire and his capacity to engage in enjoyable sex. This was completely unknown to him. Because it improves muscle mass, regular exercise can increase testosterone levels. More testosterone may be produced by the body when muscle mass increases. It is my goal to get you there since strength training becomes increasingly important as you age due to various factors, including testosterone.

James is one of many men who, like James, struggle with aging-related muscle loss, fat accumulation, and strength loss, making it difficult for them to carry out their everyday duties. When your lack of fitness prohibits you from performing tasks that you once did with ease, it can be very irritating. Unfortunately, some people believe they are too old to start exercising and that their age prevents them from building muscle or shedding fat. In actuality, you must maintain your fitness regardless of your age, and I'd even venture to suggest that it becomes even more crucial as you get older.

You are not past your prime for a workout. No of your age, maintaining a healthy weight is essential for both your physical and mental wellbeing. Your ability to manage daily tasks grows more difficult as you age, and it gets worse if you don't lead a fit lifestyle. There are several myths about the kinds of fitness activities that persons between the ages of 50 and 70 can engage in. Because of how our bodies are built, as we age, fitness may not be as heavily focused on extensive training sessions to carve off the abs. Instead, the exercises I teach are geared on keeping you in shape and reducing your risk of developing cardiovascular problems. while also enhancing your balance and muscle mass. It is crucial to be aware of your health, strength, and fitness as you reach the age of 50 and beyond.

Lack of exercise or a lack of commitment to exercise can lead to a variety of health problems. As we age, these problems grow increasingly challenging. Lack of exercise can cause muscles to stiffen, which can cause pain and discomfort when moving. Having said that, I don't want you to feel discouraged or despair over your age, lack of exercise, or irregular exercise routine after reading all of this. There is always time. Even as a young man, you can achieve a healthy, athletic lifestyle and have that amazing figure you always wanted!

I need you to do me a favor right now. Please decide consciously to act on this book's advice and give yourself the resolve to lead a healthy lifestyle. Worry less about the likelihood of getting hurt because this book's knowledge will give you all you need to train as safely as possible and put an end to injuries. The majority of the drive you require is included in this book, but the remaining portion must come from you. If you take my advise and read through each chapter, you should be well on your way to developing into the physically strong and healthy man that everyone admires. Thankfully, you don't have to do it by yourself. This book will walk you through the seven essential steps to getting the body of your dreams. I'm sure you'll have gathered a ton of knowledge you can use in your life by the time this book is up, and I'll have won your trust.

By purchasing this book, you have chosen well if you are new to fitness and strength training. Just over ten years ago, I started working as an instructor in the fitness industry. My desire is to support you in achieving all of your physical objectives. To be clear, it doesn't have to be difficult or require spending a lot of time in the gym; all you need is the willpower to persevere through the difficult parts. I put together this book because I want to assist you in doing it correctly. I have acquired information about fitness in general and, specifically, men's fitness between the ages of 40 and above via years of experience. I am aware of the enormous advantages of exercising your body and making positive changes in your life.

Okay, so now that you are familiar with me and what I have to offer, I hope you can appreciate the importance of this book. So let's get started without further ado! 5 0

U N D E R ST A N D I N G THE P O W E R O F S T R E N G T H T R A I N I N N G

You could hurt yourself if you believe that starting is useless because you missed your chance. Wrong. Opportunities will always knock on your door. It's never too late to start a practice, alter or improve a bad attitude, launch a business or career, and many other things.

Does Dwight Muhammad Qawi know you? Dwight had a fantastic career at the top of the heap despite beginning his profession at a young age in terms of boxing. At the incredibly late age of 25, Dwight eventually started participating in the sport. Even worse, he began his adventure while incarcerated in Rahway State Prison for armed robbery. As you would imagine, this man's life had reached its lowest point. The majority of individuals wouldn't anticipate him to ever achieve anything. But no matter what, there is always a path out of the shadows. He emerged from the pit of despair and went on to win world championships in the light-heavyweight and cruiserweight weight classifications. Tim Thomas, Randy Johnson, Didier Drogba, Antonio Gates, Bill Durnan, Hakeem Olajuwon, and Kurt Warner are just a few examples of sportsmen that entered their respective sports later than others but still managed to leave their impact on history. There are tens of thousands more.

Strength training definition

Strength training, as I would define it, is any physical activity intended to enhance muscular growth or fitness in a particular muscle area. It is an exercise that stresses the engaged muscles by applying a resistance force.

It entails giving your muscles more attention than they often receive. Your muscles are overworked. Any activity that targets the body's major muscular groups with a medium to high level of effort qualifies as strength training. You should be aware that strength training involves more than just using weights in a gym to bulk up. Much more is involved than that.

Older strength athletes can be broken down into three groups: those who never quit working out, those who relapsed, and those who never worked out at all. But as you become older—more over 50—strength training has indisputable advantages. Everybody can benefit from strength training, especially those with health conditions including obesity, high or low blood sugar levels, heart disease, arthritis, and many others. Strength training is an important component of the body's total fitness. Studies have demonstrated that strength training can help older adults who are physically feeble and have weak muscles.

Strength Training Methods

Strength training comes in a variety of forms, including isometric, isotonic, and isokinetic exercises. If you're still unclear as to what any of this means, don't worry. Let me clarify.

Exercises for Isometric Strength: Additionally called static strength training. Without actually extending or shortening the muscles, this sort of exercise recruits muscles and exerts stress. Your muscles are flexed, but they are not contracting or expanding. Exercises for isometric training frequently target your entire body. Additionally, it's appropriate to engage your complete body simultaneously in tasks. If you need a variation from your usual fitness regimen or have trouble with your knees, isometric exercises are a great option.

Plank and side bridge, wall sit, and other yoga postures including the chair and tree poses are all examples of isometric exercise. However, because these exercises increase strength in a single body position, they should be used in conjunction with more dynamic training programs.

Strength training that is isotonic maintains the muscle's tension or tone even as it is shortened You may think of a lot of isotonic exercises. You are purposefully extending your body across a range of motion while resisting an external weight or force. The majority of the isotonic exercise routine, including squats, pull-ups, push-ups, stair climbing, deadlifts, etc., are probably familiar to you.

Isokinetic Strength Training: This type of exercise forces you to move through a range of motion continuously. The majority of isokinetic exercise is performed on specialized machines that generate a constant force regardless of the amount of effort you put out. The equipment regulates the exercise's tempo by varying resistance over the course of your predetermined range of motion. No matter how hard you try, your speed or mobility doesn't change. You can tune the speed and range of motion to a target that best suits your requirements. Your muscular strength and endurance can be tested and enhanced through isokinetic training. Isokinetic exercise is best exemplified by using a stationary bike, which you may obtain at your neighborhood gym.

Testosterone as a Factor

Most men over 50 seem to lose their vigor, power, and energy with time. But it shouldn't be the case. The frailty and decreased energy that we frequently associate with aging include challenges with climbing, carrying burdens, and long distance walking. And each of these is mostly brought on by muscle loss. Inactivity is, in fact, one of the primary causes of muscular muscle loss. I'll give you an illustrative example. Pitch two men in their mid-50s, one who has spent years exercising and using his body, the other who spends most of his time watching old movies while seated in front of the television. Consider a situation in which you requested them to carry out a duty that they had never done before but that required some physical effort and flexibility. Who do you think does that task more effectively? The person who has consistently put effort into strength training will do better. With ease, too. You might think that this situation is apparent, but let's explore it further. First off, his body is not unfamiliar with the task and has become accustomed to performing the type of movements; second, his endurance is significantly higher, indicating that his body is well prepared to withstand the effort. This is one instance where the proverb "you either use them or lose them" applies to muscles. Your ability to perform any physical work will improve if you keep your muscles active. And by far, one of the finest methods to build those muscles is through strength training.

As we become older, testosterone levels inevitably decline in all males. A urologist at UW Health's Males's Health Clinic named David Paolone wrote in a paper that about 39% of men over the age of 45 have low testosterone. A low concentration is one that is less than 300 nanograms per deciliter. And low testosterone is more common as men age, affecting 12 percent of men in their 50s, 19 percent in their 60s, 28 percent in their 70s, and 49 percent in their 80s, according to estimates (UW Health, 2017).

Let me clarify testosterone for those who are confused. Both humans and other animals produce this hormone. The essential male sex hormone is it (also found in females but with a much lower concentration). The main source of testosterone in men is the testicles. In addition to regulating sex drive, it is essential for the development of sperm, fertility, muscle mass, bone density, fat distribution, and red blood cells. I believe you can now appreciate the significance of this hormone. During puberty, testosterone production rises, and it begins to decline beyond the age of 30. Men's testosterone levels begin to gradually decline after the age of 30 at a pace of, on average, about 1% every year. Aging naturally causes testosterone levels to decline. There are numerous effects of testosterone. When it falls below a particular level that is regarded as healthy, it might cause hypogonadism (a condition where the body doesn't generate enough male hormones or sperm) or infertility. Loss of muscular mass is a severe side effect of low testosterone.

Reduced hormone levels can cause a considerable loss of muscle because testosterone is crucial for the growth and regulation of muscle mass. Although low testosterone reduces muscular mass, it has no effect on the muscles' ability to work or their strength. Simply put, muscle mass refers to all of your body's muscles, including your skeletal, smooth, and cardiac muscles. There are risks to your health if you have low muscle mass. Your general health may suffer as a result.

Low muscle mass is linked to worse outcomes, including more post-operative and surgical problems, a longer hospital stay, decreased physical function, a lower quality of life, and shorter survival.

2021 — WITHINGS

Strength training's advantages

Many men believe that lifting weights is just useful for developing their biceps and desired six-pack. Maybe that's one of the reasons older men won't think about it. They aren't really concerned with how their body appears or how other people view them. Although I want to emphasize that this lifestyle is totally fine, strength training goes above and beyond. Strength training is crucial if you want to develop bigger biceps. Strength training is still one of the best strategies to achieve your health goals, even if reaching your maximum muscle size isn't your goal. Let me go through some of the advantages of strength training before your next workout so you can approach it and following sessions with an understanding of why you subject your body to it.

Fitness and strength.

Even though this is extremely evident, we cannot ignore it. You become fitter and stronger with strength training. Muscle strength is essential for performing daily duties, especially as you approach your fifties and naturally start to lose muscle mass. Strength training reduces the possibility of experiencing trouble carrying out daily tasks because of a lack of physical fitness. These regular activities could include stair ascending and stair descending, lifting heavy furniture or other objects, participating in sports or trekking, or even just standing still for extended periods of time. Simply said, when you're not fit and unable to perform the activities you enjoy to the best of your ability, it takes the enjoyment out of them.

protection of muscle mass and bone health.

As mentioned previously, we begin to lose an average of 1% of our lean muscle mass every year after we reach the age of 30 or so. In a 2017 study for Bone and Mineral Research, it was discovered that 30 minutes twice a week of high-intensity resistance and impact exercise increased functional performance. Additionally, postmenopausal women with poor bone mass had higher bone density, shape, and strength without experiencing any negative side effects (Watson, Weeks, Weis, Harding, Horan, Beck, 2017). Additionally, the HHS recommendations state that strength training exercises benefit everyone by maintaining or gaining muscle mass, which is important for maintaining bone, joint, and muscle health as we age (U.S. Department of Health and Human Services, 2018).

controls excessive weight

Since strength training is not centered on shedding pounds by burning as many calories as possible, it may put them off since this is a common misconception. There are a lot more types of exercise that put this first. For instance, cardiovascular exercise like running, swimming, or walking increases the amount of calories your body burns; this will definitely help you lose weight. But even if you're not burning as many calories throughout your workouts, strength training is still beneficial. Numerous studies support the idea that strength training aids in weight loss by boosting your resting metabolism. Your excess post-exercise oxygen usage rises after a successful strength training session. After a strength training session, your body keeps burning calories. Strength training keeps your metabolism going considerably longer than aerobic exercise does. In a 2017 study on "Obesity," three groups of dieters were observed: those who did no exercise, those who engaged in only aerobic activity, and those who undertook strength training activities four times per week for 18 months. Strength-training dieters dropped the most fat, on average 18 pounds. Compared to dieters who didn't exercise who only dropped 10 pounds, aerobic exercisers shed 16 pounds!

Development of Better Body Mechanics

Your posture, coordination, and balance all improve. Older persons have lower physical functioning, which increases their risk of falling. Through a strength training exercise, you can significantly lower your chance of falling. Body balance is a function of how well your stabilizing muscles are working. Your balance will be greater and steadier the more muscular you are.

Chapter 3

Osteoporosis Management and Prevention

A prevalent medical problem in older persons is osteoporosis.

The disease weakens the bones, increasing the risk of fracture. People frequently are unaware of it because it can take years to develop.

Strong bones are a feature of muscles. Your bone mineral density is considerably increased by strength training. Exercises that involve bearing weight and gravity pressing down on your body put stress on your joints and muscles. Additionally, each time a muscle contracts, it pulls on the bone that is connected to it, causing the bone cell to release structural proteins that transport minerals into the bone. Focus on standing weight-bearing exercises like lunges and squats if you want to achieve remarkable improvements in this area. Just 12 weeks of strength training with squats raised the bone mineral density of the lower spine and femur (thigh) by 2.9 and 4.9 percent, respectively, in a 2014 Journal of Family and Community Medicine study.

Control of Chronic Illnesses

The multiple advantages of strength training to treat different health problems have been well-documented in numerous research. It has been demonstrated that strength training can aid in the management of chronic illnesses. Strength training can be just as beneficial as medication at reducing arthritis pain if you have it. Strength training can help stabilize your blood sugar levels and increase how well your body uses insulin whether you have low or high blood sugar.

An increase in energy and an improvement in mood

Your endorphin levels increase when you undertake strength training, which in turn boosts your energy and elevates your mood. All workouts improve your disposition and make you feel joyful. Still, further studies on the effects of strength training on the body and how it affects the brain provides more proof that it benefits the brain (Strickland and Smith, 2014). Additionally, research suggests that strength exercise may improve your ability to sleep.

Increased Calorie Burn: Your metabolic rate is increased. Strength training increases the number of calories you burn both during and after exercise. Your body uses more energy during strength training depending on how much effort you put forth (i.e., the harder you work, the more energy is needed). Your body enters a condition of recuperation following an exercise, which causes it to burn even more calories since it requires the fuel to repair itself.

Benefits for Cardiovascular Health

Muscle-strengthening physical activity, together with aerobic exercise, helps lower blood pressure. To help lower hypertension and reduce the risk of heart illnesses, I advise you to engage in muscle-strengthening exercises twice a week in addition to 150 minutes of moderately strenuous exercise at the very least.

Greater Lifespan

The likelihood that strength training will prolong life is perhaps one of the most valuable advantages. According to a 2015 study published in The Lancet, grip strength is a reliable indicator of death from any cause. According to the study, lean muscle mass is a stronger indicator of a person's general health. A longer lifespan is directly correlated with having strong muscles.

Starting a Strength Training Program

You can be seeking for a better regimen whether you are brand-new to strength training or you have experience and are an expert at working out your body. You might fall somewhere in the middle, but you struggle to maintain consistency. In any case, let's begin your training anew, with a blank slate moving forward. Let me lead you through everything, and if you stick to my plan precisely, I can assure you that this journey will go quite smoothly. To start, you must resolve. It's simple to start something, but it takes real talent to stick with it. You must be certain of the advantages you stand to gain and, beyond that, make it a permanent attitude. It is unnecessary to be intimidated by this because, once you learn it and apply it to your life, it becomes simple, and you will find that you savor every second of it.

There are only two easy components to strength training:

any weight shifting in opposition to an opposing force Even your body weight may be a factor. Any workout that places a significant amount of stress on your muscles qualifies as strength training. overloaded gradually and doing more than before. Let's assume you began with five pushups today; after a week, you can perform six. To get stronger, your muscles will need to constantly adapt and renew.

Your strength training journey will be built on your understanding of these fundamentals.

1 The First Keey, Inc. A MIND FORTRESS

What does attitude mean? How do you put it into concrete terms so that everyone may fully comprehend it? An attitude in psychology is a person's thoughts, feelings, and actions toward a specific person, thing, or circumstance. Simply explained, attitude is an internal feeling that influences or is in charge of how we behave.

Years ago, I used an example to explain attitude to a buddy in order to show him how our attitudes influence our behavior. I questioned him about what he would do if he was driving and was struck by another car. Remember that no one was hurt, and the car suffered only minor damage. He argued back and forth for a while, attempting to understand the fictitious scenario, and then concluded that it was the right course of action for the perpetrator to be held responsible for the damages. Then I inquired as to what he would do if it transpired that I was the offender who got out of his car. This elicited a very different, warmer response, one that I must admit, I was a bit flattered by. We concluded that since he knew me and their car wasn't significantly damaged, he might let me off or accept a little settlement. Then, since we are both humans, I questioned them as to what made me different from a random criminal. They know me, which made a difference. They view me with a particular perspective or inward feeling. Your attitude alters how you approach the circumstance, which alters the result.

Every action we take depends on our mindset, so if you want to make strength training a lifestyle choice, you must have the right frame of mind. You must understand your motivation for pursuing this objective and how to maintain it. "A person cannot travel within and stand stationary without," said phycologist James Allen. The same is true in that one cannot remain motionless inside while moving outdoors. At first, this can seem unclear, so allow me to restate it. If you are unwilling to modify your views, you have little chance of succeeding in life.

It might be preferable to start by focusing on your "inward emotion." Over time, the behaviors and thoughts will eventually line up.

Allow me to assist you in developing a successful attitude and mindset for strength training.

What motivates you to exercise? It is necessary to me to question, "Why do you want to train?" Why am I doing this? is a question you should ask yourself because, in my opinion, it will make you more honest with yourself. Every time you start something new, you should start by asking yourself this straightforward question because it is crucial.

To train, you must understand why you want to. Your driving force, your initial fuel for the arduous trip ahead in life, is this question. It's one thing that will constantly support you when you're exhausted and want to give up. There is a proverb that reads, "Whenever you consider giving up, consider why you began in the first place." If you didn't have a good reason to start, then giving up at the first sign of difficulty becomes unavoidable.

That makes me think of a high school girlfriend I once had. She was a lovely girl, but she consumed an excessive amount of shit (sorry for the foul language). Although she was in good health at the moment, I wanted to help her keep it since I could tell she was going in the wrong direction. I begged her repeatedly to accompany me to the gym so we could both check it out. She finally agreed to try it after much persuasion in an effort to silence me. If I said our relationship was flawless, I would be lying. Over time, I came to the realization that a girl's good looks are irrelevant if she makes you miserable. As you might have guessed, we parted ways after five months of dating. Ironically, I never again ran into her in that gym. And while it's possible that she didn't want to deal with our awkward hallway encounters, I really believe it was due to her lack of conviction. She left because she thought I would want anything, and after I was gone, she was left with nothing.

You must be personally persuaded to exercise: Alright, so now you may be asking yourself, "What's the best motivation to exercise?" In actuality, there isn't one. Because we are all different, everyone has distinct motivations. Your conviction may be fueled by several things. It could be one of the advantages we discussed in chapter one. You may use it as a means of escaping reality and spending your time on worthwhile activities. It may even be as easy as you just want to show off your toned six pack to all girls you encounter. Make sure that everything that would strengthen your conviction is for you and not merely a means of stopping someone from complaining. My friend, as soon as you decide, we can move on. Let's continue...

Your belief gives you the self-motivation you need to start a new endeavor. If you begin this trip and find it challenging to fulfill that pledge each day, don't worry. When you do anything enough times, your brain plays a cute little trick on you that goes like this: you want to do something fairly difficult; you start with the small bit of drive you have only to discover the more you do it, the easier it gets. Your brain develops a little area that alerts you when it's time to perform a task because you consistently perform the same task. The best thing is that every time you complete that activity, your brain releases dopamine, also known as the "feel-good" hormone, as a reward.

Make time for training: Strength training instructor Bobby Maximus stated, "One of the main challenges people face when it comes to training is finding adequate time. Much of the training conversation focuses on exercise and diet. The main factor in a person's success in any given training program appears to be time management.

I don't want to prejudge whether you have a lot of time or none at all. Sincerity dictates that it is irrelevant. The adage "if you want something bad enough, you'll find a way; if not, you'll find an excuse" comes to me when

I think about time. Also, I think you'll find time for it if it's essential to you. After considering the advantages of exercising and deciding why you want to do this, it's time to make time—even if we have to create it out of thin air. "I've coached many different types of people with differing levels of commitment," continued Bobby Maximus. I am often dissatisfied with how much time people are willing to provide. So let me be clear: lack of time is not an excuse. Usually, a person's lack of commitment or poor time management skills are the real problem.

Let me assist you if time management is what's getting in your way. Everyone day has 24 hours for each of us. This time is ours to do with as we like. You may easily set aside roughly three hours per week for your training if you have excellent time management skills. You'll find the time you never imagined you had if you use the guide I've created below to manage your priorities:

High Priority/High Urgency These are prioritized over all else.

High Importance/Low Urgency: You can order these projects and fit them into your day, working on tiny portions at a time, or you can set deadlines to complete them. Low Importance/High Urgency: You should find quick, effective ways to complete this assignment without involving yourself too much personally. Make a plan for things in advance to get them done as quickly as you can.

Low Priority: These are time-consuming or repetitive operations, like filling. Stack them up and complete everything at once each week, have someone else do them, or skip it altogether.

To maximize your productivity at work, schedule your week keeping this in mind.

Prioritize while beginning: What is speed? Velocity is simply speed plus direction. Ensure that you are aware of the distinction between velocity and speed. When your focus is absent, speed is worthless. It's the same as starting a strength training program without a purpose. You must choose your objectives and set goals.

Without goals, it is impossible to gauge your progress, and you risk becoming worn out and exhausted at any time. Additionally, setting up clear milestones will increase motivation each time you reach one of them. Proven success is one of the best motivators, so take advantage of it.

Obtain social assistance

People frequently undervalue and ignore the use of social assistance. For novices and even seasoned trainers looking for individuals to share their achievement with, social support from other males undergoing a strength training program may be a great windfall. It is much simpler to express feelings, questions, problems, and accomplishments when you are around by people who share your viewpoints. You won't fail or lose heart if you have the help of people who are in a similar situation to yourself because the group won't let you!

Although there are various methods to join a group, it might be a little frightening to contact new individuals directly. Joining a community on social media is a terrific method to get around this. I suggest using Facebook. There are hundreds of groups here that share your objectives among millions of groups from around the world. It's easy to join them; all you have to do is enter your search term in the search bar. A wonderful alternative if you're not a social media guy is to join a gym where you can make connections with other older men for social support. You'll realize you're not alone because of others' hardships.

However, their success stories can give you motivation and reassurance that your aim of starting a strength training regimen is attainable. It will dispel any uncertainty you might have regarding strength training. I implore you to recognize the value of friendship.

Additionally, you might workout as a group or even hold friendly tournaments to enliven and ignite the group's desire. Studies have demonstrated that competitive games encourage people to work more. I can definitely relate to that. Friends have warned me that I occasionally become a little too competitive (especially in board games).

When uncertainty sets in, the truth is that you could grow weary along the way. With all the effort, you can find yourself getting worn out or not achieving the expected outcomes. Although it may be easy, giving up is the worst course of action when you believe you are not obtaining the intended outcomes. Take a moment, look over your plan, and make sure you aren't expecting too much in a short amount of time or an unexpected outcome. People frequently make this mistaken assumption, but I want you to realize that life is a marathon, not a sprint. You must be ready for the long hall and handle everything with grace. Reduce the weight you're training with, the quantity of repetitions, or the amount of sets if you're in pain. Moving slowly and gradually is preferable to moving quickly and burning out.

Don't assess yourself against others: "Comparison is a thief of joy," goes a proverb. You can discover yourself in one of the following circumstances: When you run into your friend who started around the same time as you and realize that he has made more progress than you have, you start to feel irritated and disheartened. You have been following your workout plan religiously and seeing benefits along the way, which makes you feel good. And while you were content with yourself only a second ago, everything disappears as you see something better.

Social comparison is common in some cases. According to some studies, evaluating how you stack up against others can be a powerful motivator. Messages about what one should aspire to in our culture abound, but sadly, these messages are not always logical or achievable. We contrast apples and oranges rather than apples and apples.

The man you are contrasting yourself with because of his toned abs most likely inherited a different body type from you, making it easier for him to gain muscle or burn fat. People frequently use filters to make the pictures and success stories they post online and offline look ideal. You could feel like a failure and lose confidence in yourself if you make frequent, irrational comparisons between yourself and others. Additionally, the comparison makes you feel like you are not accomplishing enough because it makes you concentrate more on others than on yourself. Keep in mind that this adventure is only for you. You start an internal emotion that might develop into anxiety and self-doubt when you start wondering that you won't have what the other guy has. Additionally, comparing yourself to others might harm your friendships and your connections with your workout partners. It is nearly impossible to support one another and really celebrate when you hit milestones when you are jealous of one another's successes.

Variety should be included in your training.

It might get monotonous and exhausting to keep doing the same thing over and over. To add some entertainment to your training, you must spice up your approach. Our brains are wired to want variety. If you have been exercising the same way over and over, you should think about stretching. Consider some unconventional concepts that appeal to you and seem secure. Maybe you should pick up a sport as a hobby. Look for a company where you can hire kayaks and local outdoor groups where you may go kayaking with others. Make sure that everything you choose to do in this regard is safe for you.

Give yourself some time to acclimate to the recent activities your body is suffering, even if your new routine isn't particularly hard.

Exercise discipline

Although most of us are generally aware of the idea of discipline, very few of us actually get what it means. Every day, successful people practice discipline. We all depend on it, and without it, everything would be in disarray. A form of freedom is self-discipline, which includes freedom from lethargy and sloth, from other people's demands and expectations, from attempting to please other people at the price of your own convenience, from doubts and worries, from fast pleasure, and many other things. You must exercise discipline if you want to train efficiently and get the best results. To resist something you crave takes a lot of strength. It also requires plenty of discipline to carve out time to train and be consistent with yourself.

Be persistent

Mike Boyle once compared training to farming in his analogy. You do action today that you don't view as having an impact in the anticipation of a reward down the road. To increase the likelihood that some little green shoots may eventually emerge from the earth, you sow the seeds, provide water and fertilizer, and frighten away the birds.

The results take time to manifest; you can't sow a seed now and expect to see a crop tomorrow. The same is true of strength training. It requires time. People who haven't seen you in a while start complimenting you on how terrific you look and asking if you've lost weight once these shoots begin to appear. You might not see any noticeable changes after a month or two of daily self-examination, but persistence and consistency will eventually provide results. You feel better, your muscles are easier to see, and you get faster, stronger, and more physically fit. And things seem to be getting a little better.

Expense yourself

Anything with a significant payoff is completed by someone. Do you know why people perform a variety of professions rather than all of us performing the same task, especially those that are quite taxing? Take garbage collectors as an illustration. As I'm sure you are all aware, a garbage collector's responsibility is to travel around the designated region and gather rubbish, whether it be for residential, commercial, industrial, or other purposes. A tough stomach is needed for this somewhat thankless work, if you know what I mean. So why would someone volunteer their time to perform such a challenging task? It's because they receive a comparatively generous wage. Depending on where they work, garbage collectors in the UK can make up to £45,000 a year. All they need is a high school diploma, which is equivalent to $62,500 in the United States. Regardless of the work itself, there will never be a scarcity of waste collectors at these wages. Being rewarded for your efforts is a strong motivator and motivation. I want you to employ this effective motivation the next time you achieve a goal, no matter how minor. I can guarantee that if you treat yourself by doing something you enjoy, your motivation will soar.

Using money as an incentive increases people's likelihood to exercise and maintain consistency for up to six months or even longer, according to a study of 11 randomized research involving roughly 1,500 participants. Additionally, the effectiveness is influenced by the design of the financial incentives. In a study, researchers set the daily step goal for 280 participants to be 7,000. The participants were divided into one of four groups at random: the first group received $1.40 for every 7,000 steps they took each day, which amounted to $42 in a month; the second group had a chance to win $1.40 in a lottery prize each day; the third group received $42 up front with $1.40 deducted for each day they did not reach 7,000 steps; and the fourth group served as a control group with no incentive. After 13 weeks, the team that had received money up front emerged victorious. The fact that losing $1.40 every day posed a greater incentive than the prospect of earning it is noteworthy. This characteristic is referred to by economists and decision theorists as "loss aversion": We detest losing money even more than we despise receiving it.

How can you use this method to inspire yourself? Giving money to someone you trust to manage your money on a regular basis is one approach to do this. You receive your money back for each month you attend your gym sessions consistently, which you can then use to reward yourself with a trip or other purchase you've been wanting to make. However, if you don't show up, the person who is in possession of your money gives it to your wife or children as pocket money. Or you could create your own method. Whatever method you use, it works well as a motivator when there is an incentive involved.

Hopefully, you now have a better understanding of the mental toughness needed to set out on this adventure. It will initially require some willpower, but if you can get through the early storm, a sunny day is waiting for you.

Chapter 4

BUILDING YOUR FOUNDATIONS: THE SECONDDKEY

If you plan to construct a home, the first thing you need do is sit down and calculate the cost to determine whether you have enough money to pay for the entire project. You will end yourself in a position where the house cannot be built and you have lost all of your time if you fail to take this stage seriously and proceed through the procedure with care and attention. The phrase "This man started to create and was unable to complete" may be used.

The Bible records the words of Jesus Christ, which are those said above. It doesn't matter if you follow Jesus

Christ or not. Beginning at the very beginning of the trip is where success begins. You're starting a strength training program and want to stick with it until the end since following through on a plan gives you a lot of happiness. It advances you and inspires you to accomplish more.

Although it is impossible, many beginners would love to have insight into their program, be able to predict how well they will progress, or even wish to have made some progress already. A journey does not begin in the middle. You begin at the beginning and are subject to what is in store for you.

The numerous difficult queries that will wish to keep you from ever starting in the first place are one of the issues you can experience prior to taking your first steps. Such inquiries as "Can I do this? How will this affect how others perceive me? What if I have to make a large purchase? Can I make sense of this? You might become paralyzed by all of these concerns and perhaps hesitate to begin your strength training regimen.

This is why it's so important to calculate the cost up front. By calculating the cost of starting a new pastime, you may create a plan for the future. By providing guidance, blueprints assist in providing answers to challenging questions. They enable you to fill in the minor details and perceive the overall picture. A blueprint gives you the assurance that, if you follow each step, you will get the desired outcome. the belief that there is a tried-and-true way to get from point A to point B. You'll have a better chance of success if you stick to the laid out plan rather than strike off on your own. I'm here to provide you with whatever you need to get going because of this. Just be careful not to disregard this plan, which was carefully and attentively created for you like a house.

What are the requirements to begin your training?

Many might advise you to begin by hiring a personal coach. However, the majority of people don't have the time or resources to do so.

However, if you desire to get some fancy new toys, you can do so with the following equipment but just remember, it's not necessary:

Dumbbells

We all know about these. They are the well-known fitness equipment. If you are new to strength training, dumbbells are an excellent place to start. Dumbbells are short bars with weights at each end. It can be used individually using a higher weight or in pairs simultaneously. Mostly all gyms are equipped with dumbbells ranging from 1kg to 50kg. If used properly, they're easy on your joints and great for developing strength. Because your hands are not fixed in place, they allow your body to move organically. I'll advise you to get adjustable dumbbells. This will allow you to add weights as you progress in your program. A beginner's set of 10kg adjustable weight dumbbells goes for an average of $50 - the price increases when you add more weight, understandably.

Barbells

Barbells are not just for athletes competing in a competition. Being the big brother to dumbbells, they can be lifters' friends for moves like deadlifts, back squats, and snatches. A barbell is like the longer, two-handed form of a dumbbell. It's a long metal bar to which weights are attached at each end. You can decide on the weight if it's an adjustable barbell, just like dumbbells. They allow you to add much more weight than dumbbells due to the strength of the bar. You can have as high as 20kg plates on each side of the metal bar. It would be best if you considered the weight of the metal bar too. Going between 15kg to 25kg is fair for you at the start. Do not purchase fixed barbells because you want to increase weight when training you progressively. Barbells are pretty expensive. An adjustable 50kg barbell could go for $200 on average so maybe save up a bit for that one. Remember, they are by no means necessary, and I will teach you workouts that don't require any equipment later on in this book.

Kettlebells

They are cannonball-like weights with a single loop handle. It's almost like the shape of a kettle, except it's got no spout. Like kettlebell swings and cleans, many classic kettlebell exercises require you to quickly and powerfully exert force on the weight. It's also a great way to work in some heart-pumping cardio. The weight of the kettlebell isn't balanced like a dumbbell; it shifts as you move it, this makes your body work harder to stabilize. It's excellent for training your balance. Considering you're over 50, kettlebells are great because they teach your body to adapt to the changing center of gravity. Just try not to fall over; I've made that mistake before. A 15kg kettlebell could go for $70 on average. Electric kettlebells, which are adjustable, are expensive and could go for over $250 on average.

Body Bars

The body bar is one of the simplest to use of all the strength training equipment, yet it is probably one of the least well-known. It's a slender long metal pole covered in foam rubber. It ranges in weight, making it a friendlier (and lighter weight) alternative to standard barbells. Body bars let you perform all kinds of exercises that you use barbells for, and they can be a good start for beginners. I recommend a 10kg body bar if you are a complete beginner. They are sold at around $50.

TRX\sTRX stands for total body resistance exercise. It's a single piece of equipment made from two nylon straps suspended from the ceiling. You can use TRX to perform hundreds of strength training exercises, from push-ups to planks. TRX is an all-in-one tool. One of its most prominent benefits is dynamicity and versatility instead of an isolated movement. You will be working multiple muscle groups all at once. For instance, you can slip your feet into the TRX handles; your regular push-up turns into a core and shoulder-stabilizing move. And because you're using your body weight, you can adjust the resistance by moving your feet further (more resistance) or closer (less resistance) away from the anchor point. TRX could go for $40 on average.

Medicine Balls

They look a little like basketballs, but I don't think you could throw them that far. They are weighted balls, roughly the diameter of your shoulders. It's called a medicine ball because it also plays a vital role in sports medicine to improve strength and neuromuscular coordination. This ball-shaped weight can add resistance to core exercises like Russian twists or sit-ups. You can also carry, lift or throw it. Moving medicine balls in several directions and planes of motion can involve more tissue, which helps lift energy use. A medicine ball could go for $25 on average.

Stability Balls

They are inflatable beach-ball-like strength training tools. They are helpful for bodyweight exercises that focus on the primary muscle that attaches the pelvis to the femurs (thigh bone) and spine. They can help you increase and improve spine stability through moves like back extensions and planks. This is very good for you if you spend a lot of time sitting at a desk. A 60cm stability ball could go for $15 on average.

Slam Balls

They are just like medicine balls. Although they are slightly larger and sometimes heavier, they don't bounce. It means you don't need to worry about the ball jumping into your face after you slam it. You can use slam balls to develop power, speed, and strength. Your muscles respond in proportion to how fast and powerful you slam the ball. A 10kg slam ball could go for $10 on average.

Resistance Bands

Resistance bands look like giant rubber bands. They are either flat or tubular. The different types of resistance bands may confuse you, but they fall under the same category. Although, they are used differently. They provide an effective workout. They are low impact and joint-friendly. Because the band creates resistance in both directions, your body is forced to remain stable. It will help you in training for balance. You can choose your desired resistance level, style, and length. You'll find everything from flat bands to tube bands with handles or even closed-looped bands. Try to get accustomed to their tension; at first, they might seem a little awkward, but you will get the hang of them over time. Resistance bands are perfect for exercises like squats, overhead press, and lateral band walks. This equipment is easy to move around, so you could even take them with you if you travel. Resistance bands are minimal in design and made out of cheap material, so you can typically get your hands on some for $15.

Sandbags

Just as the name describes, sandbags are weighted bags of sand; they look like big duffle bags. They are handy strength training tools made of durable materials. You can fill various materials inside them, not just sand. The materials you fill are known as fillers, and they're used for multiple functions while training. Although most people fill with sand, you can use pea gravel and rubber mulch. It's the best sandbag filler, in my opinion, because they don't make dust or pulverize. You can push your sandbag up, slam them down and slide them across the floor like a champ. Or, incorporate them into your strength training routine via squats, lunges, and carries. Sandbags will help improve functional fitness and get you ready for daily activities like carrying kids, bags of groceries, moving furniture, etc. And because the sand shifts as you move the bag, it helps challenge your wrist and forearm muscles, making them work harder to control the movement of the weight. Be sure not to fill your bag with more than 10kg for a start. Increase the fill as you progress in your training. You can get a moderate size sandbag for $10 on average.

ViPR

ViPR stands for vitality, performance, and reconditioning. ViPR is used to bridge the gap between movement and strength training. It combines full-body movement with load; hence, the name. ViPR builds mobility, stability, and dynamic strength through loaded movement training. Since you can pick it up and shift it in space, it mimics movements in sport and forces your body to work together. You can make forward lunges with rotation or lateral lunges while you swing the ViPR over and up as if you're using a shovel to dig. The ViPR can help you improve the strength and resilience of muscles and tissues, making it more resistant to many kinds of stain injuries. The muscles become lengthened under resistance and enhance the tissue's strength and density. The intensity of the movement can be altered based on how you hold the ViPR and how you move the tool to your center of mass. Pushing it further from your body makes it more challenging. ViPRs are pretty expensive... A 10kg ViPR could go for $200 on average. But don't worry, none of my teachings involve using these.

BOSU Balance Trainer

It is also referred to as a BOSU ball. BOSU stands for both sides utilized, which means you can use both the dome stability ball-like side and the flat side for exercises. It is like a stability ball cut in half. It consists of an inflated rubber hemisphere attached to a rigid platform. It is mainly used for balance training. You can use the dome side for exercises such as crunches on a softer surface that allows the full range of motion of the spine. You can stand on the flat surface to create a unique balance platform that helps engage lower body muscles. It's also perfect for building dynamic balance, enabling you to balance while in motion or change positions. A BOSU balance trainer could go for over $150 on average.

Gliding Discs

They are small, flat, two-sided round discs; one side is a fabric, and the other is hard plastic, or depending on your choice, both sides may have canvas-like material. You can use them on your feet and hands to provide a smooth gliding surface. Use these plate-size discs to crank up reverse or lateral lunges. You are sure to feel your core, glutes and inner thighs light up. They are also great for ab exercises like mountain climbers and pikes. Since you take resistance away from your feet, your core has to do all the work of stabilizing your body. A pair of gliding discs could go for only $10, so it's a good investment.

Parallettes

They are gymnastic tools, which are used in pairs. They are used to simulate the parallel bars found in professional gymnasiums. Much like push-up bars or dip bars, they are generally longer and lower to the ground. Gymnasts commonly use them. Parallettes allow you to test the limit of your physical strength. They allow you to perform exercises such as handstand push-ups, L-sits, and other gnarly feats of strength. And since you are raised off the ground, you can move into a deeper range of motion with each exercise. Parallettes could go for $60 on average, which isn't bad if you ask me.

Battle Ropes

If you want a hard and grueling workout, consider a workout with combat ropes. Battle ropes are used for fitness training to increase fullbody strength and conditioning. They may not seem like much at first glance, but they provide a fantastic workout. Grab the rope with two hands and start lifting up and down to create waves or hold them in different hands for a more incredible exercise. The bigger the wave, the more energy you're putting into the rope. Try to keep the ropes moving fast. Using battling rope is like doing sprints for your upper body. Due to the fact that you must continually apply force to the lifts to maintain the wave pattern, they are ideal for addressing balance concerns. Battle ropes could go for $40 on average.

The equipment listed above is all acceptable if you desire to have your strength training workout at home. Several of the items on the list can be added to your home gym. I recommend using a body bar, resistance band, dumbbell, and possibly a TRX. The figures listed above are only an estimate of what it might cost you on average. The brand of any equipment you're buying has a significant impact on prices.

Also keep in mind that you can join a gym to gain complete access to a wider variety of equipment, including exercise machines. However, because fixed exercise devices like smith machines limit your body's natural movements, I do not recommend them.

Chapter 5

ADVICE FOR NEWCOMERS

Warm-Up

Since you are over 50 and have never worked out previously, it's likely that your muscles are unaccustomed to resistance exercise. You'd be so much better off doing some cardio workouts. You could help your muscles get ready by engaging in brisk walking or jogging for a day or two. Your muscles will receive more blood as a result, which will get them ready for an effective workout.

Start off slowly

Start lifting weights at a weight that you can do at least five to eight times while maintaining perfect form. Start with one or two sets of 5–8 repetitions and work your way up over time. Everyone has to start somewhere, so no one will make fun of you for utilizing a lighter weight.

use appropriate form

The proper form must be used when exercising. Use your joints' entire range of motion when lifting weights. Slowly and deliberately doing the exercise will increase the strain you place on your muscles. The better your form, the better the outcome, and the less likely it is that you will get hurt. Decrease the weight or the number of repetitions if you can't keep your form.

Between-Workout Rest: Resting in between workouts helps beginners avoid muscle exhaustion. Additionally, when lifting, try not to hold your breath. When lifting the weight, exhale, and when lowering it, inhale.

Spend no more than 20 minutes working out: At first, don't go overboard. Though you could still feel like you're in your 30s, you need to take your age into account. You'll get good results in twenty minutes. You can eventually raise it to 30 minutes.

Observe any soreness

Do not continue working out if you have pain; stop right away. Try the workout again in a few days, or try using lighter weights.

Rest

Before the following session, resting allows your muscles to heal and restock their energy reserves.

Clothing

Without sufficient protection, you cannot exercise. Get workout-appropriate footwear and gloves.

How to be safe while strength training

When strength training, you need to have the proper form and body positioning. You run the risk of hurting yourself if you perform some of these exercises incorrectly. Although the exercises in the book include visuals to go with them, if you're confused about your technique, you may check out training videos online.

You can increase the weight by roughly 5% once you get used to lifting that particular weight. But never rush a situation. Building is the aim, not getting hurt. Do your best to stay secure.

3-Thirds of the Kingdom Elite Bodyweight Exercise Each day, more and more of our muscular mass is lost.

Physical fitness reduces as we age. more so when we age over 50. In particular, testosterone levels drop, weight usually rises, and the likelihood of being sick or catching a disease significantly increases. The main strategies for preventing the unavoidable impacts of aging include regular exercise, especially strength training, adequate nutrition, and nutritional supplements.

One of the main goals of your strength training program should be to prevent injuries, poor balance, and bad posture. This chapter will include bodyweight workouts that you may perform at home without any special equipment. A fitness exercise that doesn't include a machine or external weight may raise some doubts in the minds of certain people. However, studies have shown that bodyweight exercises increase strength and stamina. They are safe exercises that anyone can perform whenever they choose. Finding enough exercises to create an entire routine seems to be the biggest challenge people confront. Don't worry; I've put up a list of all of my top selections that targets every muscle area for you.

BODYWEIGHT TRAINING

Bodyweight exercises are straightforward strength training routines that rely on your own weight to defy gravity. They are efficient methods for enhancing one's strength, balance, power, flexibility, endurance, speed, etc. without the stress of having to purchase and acquire the necessary equipment. Simple movements like pulling, squatting, twisting, pushing, and balancing are used in bodyweight training. Pull-ups, push-ups, and sit-ups are a few of the common bodyweight exercises, but there are many more.

If you're still unsure, consider some of the advantages listed below that come without utilizing weights or other tools.

Convenient: While using weights for exercise has advantages, utilizing your body weight is more practical than using dumbbells or barbells. Anywhere you are, whether inside or outside, you can get a heart-pumping and efficient workout using your hands and feet.

Efficient: Since there is no TRX, kettlebell, or ViPR in the way, you can switch between moves quickly. Your heart rate stays raised when you sleep less, which is crucial for burning calories. Interval training is frequently used for bodyweight exercises; you alternate between short bursts of intensive effort and slower or no activity intervals. It has been shown that this is more effective than continuous cardio.

Squats and push-ups are among the most versatile exercises. Both movements are compound. They focus on the most noticeable muscle groups and include several joints.

Customizable: Bodyweight exercises provide you a wide range of alternatives for any fitness level whereas equipment has limitations. It merely requires finding them. The push-up, for instance, can be performed in a variety of forms, from knees on the ground to clap and handstand variations.

Free: Although you can perform a bodyweight workout in a gym, all you need is a flat surface; therefore, you can perform it at home without spending any money on equipment.

THE FINAL STAGE OF BODYWEIGHT ACTIVITIES.

I hope by now you realize the value of your own flesh. Let's get started with the workouts I believe to be the greatest of the best. I'll be going through these exercises, their advantages, and how to perform them properly. They have all been specifically picked for your age range with the goal of preventing injuries. Using only a small amount of information on a page, it can be challenging to visualize the proper arrangement of an exercise. I have included examples of each action that contains a starting position and a finishing position to get around this. Because they are numbered, you can always look them up and use them as a reference.

Leg strengthening exercises will be performed first.

1. SQUAT

A squat is a strength workout in which you keep your back straight while lowering your hip from a standing position. Your hip and knee joints flex as you lower yourself to squat, while your ankles dorsiflex (flexion of the ankle upwards). In contrast, when you stand up, your ankle joints plantarflex (stretch downward) and your hip and knee joints extend. Squats come in a variety of forms, but to keep things straightforward, we'll only talk about the common squat. How to exercise:

Pose: You should be in the correct squat stance before you squat. Maintain a small gap between your feet and shoulders. Rather than pointing straight forward, they should be angled out between 5 and 30 degrees, depending on your level of comfort. This aids in maintaining balance. Maintain a firm foundation: Your muscles will be more actively used, your alignment will be better, and you'll be more stable on the ground if you plant your feet firmly. Furthermore, it will prevent your arches from collapsing.

Put your chest up: Your upper body is also important. You must roll your shoulders back and keep your chest high. Imagine an invisible pole running from the back of your head to your lower back.

starting the movement You should begin a squat by bending your knees and pushing your hips back when you're ready to do so. As you lower, brace your core and keep it there throughout the bend. Throughout the entire movement, make sure to maintain control and go slowly. Your muscles will be under tension for a longer period of time as a result, working harder. Inhale as you lower yourself, and as you squat, make sure your knees are lateral to your toes and not too inward or outward.

I advise pointing your arms directly in front of you for added stability if you're seeking for anything to do with them.

When you come to a right angle, stop. To add resistance, you can bend more deeply, but as long as you stop when your legs are at a straight angle, it's acceptable. It is preferable to stop the exercise at any point where it is comfortable and pain-free for you if you are having trouble reaching there owing to limited mobility or an injury. While standing, push through your heels: Throughout the entire squat, make sure your feet are planted firmly on the ground. When rising back up, concentrate on pressing through your heels. Your hamstrings and glutes, which are located in the back of your body, will get a boost of energy from this. It would be better if you let out a breath as you climbed back up.

Always remember to breathe, inhale on the way down and exhale on the way up.

2. LUNGE

Have you ever seen a football player on the field of play bend down to re-tie a shoelace? If someone makes a kneeling proposal, you are likely familiar with the lunge. A single-leg bodyweight exercise called a lunge targets your hips, quadriceps, glutes, hamstrings, and inner thighs. Lunges can increase lower body strength and endurance. When performed correctly, they efficiently target the muscles in your lower body without adding to the load on your joints. They are excellent starter moves.

How to work out:

One of your legs should be in front of the other as you stand in a split stance. Take one stride forward or one step backward to reach the correct length.

Before you lunge, make sure your torso is straight and that you are on your toes waiting for the rear leg.

When you simultaneously bend both knees, squat down until your back knee is 3 to 4 inches off the ground. The floor should be parallel to the front thigh. Both of your legs should bear the same amount of your weight.

Straighten your front leg to push yourself back up. Before switching legs, repeat each rep.

Your knees may suffer a great deal from lunges. They can ease the strain of lunges by implementing the following advice:

Keep your entire front leg foot firmly planted on the ground.

Keep in mind that doing a lunge relies on your hips. Maintain a squared-off posture with your hip bones facing front for more balanced joint and muscle exercise.

The rib cage should always be above the pelvis since doing so will promote improved posture and muscle engagement. Avoid raising your ribcage. It could put strain on your low back. You will breathe easier and exert more force when your rib cage is over your pelvis. Your toes and front knee should be in correct alignment. Lunges must be performed properly for joint health.

You may want to think about the side lunge as an alternative or for diversity. Standing straight up and shoulder-width apart is a good place to start. Step out to the side as far as you can while maintaining a straight back. Push back up to the starting position after lowering until the knee of your leading leg is bent at about 90 degrees while keeping your trailing leg straight. Collapsing over the straight knee may be a problem with the side lunge. Keep your back straight and your core tight, exactly like you would when performing a squat, and concentrate on bending and descending from the hips. Last but not least, be careful to maintain a flat foot.

GLUTE BRIDGE 3.

A versatile, taxing, and efficient bodyweight exercise is the glute bridge. The glute bridge is a great supplement to any exercise program, regardless of your age or level of fitness. It targets your glutes and hamstrings.

How to work out:

On the floor or an exercise mat, lie on your back. With both of your feet flat on the ground, bending your knees. Put your knees, feet, and shoulders in line. Flatten your lower back into the floor by contracting your abdominal muscles. Try to keep your back straight throughout the workout.

Gently exhale as you pass your hips upward off the floor into extension and focus your core. When you reach full extension, pinch your bottom. To increase stability, make sure your feet are firmly planted on the ground. Avoid raising your hips too much because doing so will likely cause your low back to arch more.

As you gradually lower yourself back into your starting position, take a breath.

Make progress gradually with this exercise. You can switch to the single-leg glute bridge after performing several repetitions with both feet on the floor. To prevent arching your lower back, keep your hips from being raised too high.

The single-leg glute bridge is performed by lying on your back while bending your knees until your feet are flat on the ground, as previously mentioned. Next, lift and straighten one of your legs. Drive your hips up while maintaining a straight leg in the air, and then perform the glute bridge as usual.

FIRE HYDRANT 4.

As well known as hip abductions on quadrupeds. It is a bodyweight workout that targets the gluteus maximus in particular, however some forms can also target the core. Hip extension, hip external rotation, and hip abduction are the three main hip movements regulated by the glutes. All three actions are performed by the fire hydrant. You'll get steely buns if you do this consistently. A good set of glutes will help you stand straighter, experience less back and knee pain, and experience less chance of injury.

How to work out:

You begin by standing on your hands and legs. as if crawling, with your hands under your shoulders and your legs beneath your hips. Keep your knees hip-width apart at all times.

Maintain a flat back, level hips, a tight core, and 90-degree bent legs. As you extend your leg, bring it to hip height and hold it there for a brief period of time.

To put the leg back in its original position, lower it. After many repetitions, switch to the other leg.

Be sure to keep your back straight and face the floor. Keep your elbows locked and resist the urge to transfer your weight to one side. Take your time, and avoid putting your leg higher than your hip. As you lift and drop your leg, take a breath in and out.

STEP UP 5.

You have to step up to a higher level and then step back down, as the name would imply. Stepping up is a straightforward body resistance exercise that tones your bottom and leg muscles. The quadriceps muscles at the front of the thigh are strengthened as a result. It's a terrific technique to balance this out because walking and running seldom activate the quadriceps. Developing your quads will also keep your knees safe. As long as you have a sturdy surface to walk on, like a bench, you may execute the step-up exercise anyplace.

How to work out:

Use a step around you or a box or chair as a support while you are standing there. Initially, using the stairs at home is acceptable, but keep in mind that the resistance increases with step height. You will eventually need to upgrade to something taller.

While the other is down, put one of your feet up on the step.

To straighten the leg, push through your heel.

Bring the second foot to rest against the step's top foot.

Step down with the opposite foot after bending the first knee on the step.

Bring down the step's other foot as well.

Any number of times can be done, then switch sides and lead with the opposite foot as you go through the motions again.

6. CALF RAISE

Most people try to disregard their calves, but you don't want to be the guy who puts on his shorts and looks like a popsicle stick, do you? It doesn't look good. They play a crucial role in your day-to-day activities. Consider the activities of walking or running. For inactive people, calf muscles might be stiff due to a lack of flexibility. Consider warming up by performing a little walking to let your calf muscles relax. The gastrocnemius and soleus muscles, which run along the back of the lower leg, are engaged during the calf raise. Running and jumping are made possible by these muscles, which are essential for ankle flexion and extension. Additionally, the gastrocnemius and hamstrings collaborate to govern knee flexion. In order to keep the body balanced, the soleus pumps blood from the legs to the heart. Running and walking become challenging when the calf muscles are weak because they are susceptible to cramping and strain.

How to work out:

Place your feet shoulder-width apart and steadily lift your heels while maintaining an extended knee position. Hold your position on your toes for a little moment.

Returning your heels to the ground carefully.

On the basis of science and study, those are my top recommendations for the lower body. Let's now go on to strengthening your core.

CRUNCH 7.

One traditional core workout is the crunch. It is a fantastic compound-muscle exercise for the abdominals. It exercises your upper and lower abdominal, oblique, and lower back muscles when done properly. Your entire body is stabilized by these muscles. Crunches assist you build your stabilizing muscles, such as the spinal erector muscles, as well as get a toned, ripped stomach (your back). There are other advantages for the stomach as well; by causing bowel spasms and causing it to move, it aids those who from regular constipation. You can burn a lot of calories just a few minutes of moderate crunches. The burn you get when exercising the core is, however, my personal favorite aspect. You'll come to adore it!

How to work out:

On the ground, lie on your back. (An workout mat would be better because it is more pleasant.)

Place your feet level on the ground while raising your knees and bending them. Hip width should be the distance between the knees and the feet. The distance between your heels and tailbone should be around a foot and a half.

On your chest, cross both arms. If it makes you feel more at ease, you can also place your fingertips behind your head or neck.

In a smooth, controlled motion, raise your shoulder blades off the mat. Breathe in, then exhale while contracting your abdominal muscles and raising your torso. Just enough lifting is required to get your shoulder blades off the floor. Once lifted, hold the position for a few seconds. (You can suffer lower back discomfort if you elevate your entire torso off the floor). Make sure the floor is in contact with your feet, tailbone, and lower back.

Lower yourself back slowly and steadily. Gently inhale as you slowly lower your torso. Moving with smooth control will work your abs more efficiently and help you stay injury-free. Always take a brief break between reps. Rushing the next rep can cause you to exhaust yourself by lifting yourself rather than your muscles, which could result in back injury. The trick is to picture your abs just raising your body. Keeping them tense throughout the motion is beneficial.

Eight. FLUTTER KICK

The flutter kick is a workout that targets your core muscles. It primarily targets the hip flexors and the lower rectus abdominal muscles. You can do this exercise by lying on your back (or stomach if you want to build your back muscles) and utilizing your core to flutter your legs back and forth, similar to swimming strokes. Flutter kicks increase endurance, balance, and posture as well as aid to prevent injuries. Additionally, it can aid in calorie burning and give abs with more definition.

How to work out:

Lay flat on your back while angling your legs at a 45-degree angle. Put your arms behind your butt or keep them straight with the floor. You can raise a small portion of your shoulders, neck, and head off the ground.

Start by lowering one leg while keeping your legs straight and fastened to one another.

Focusing on maintaining an engaged core, raise the lowered leg and lower the other.

Keep switching back and forth between the two legs.

Russian Twist 9.

The Russian twist is the last exercise in our core routine. This beneficial workout gives you a toned midsection and a stronger back by strengthening all of your abdominal muscles, as well as your internal and external obliques. The key to this technique is the twisting motion. A common workout among athletes, it promotes rotational mobility, an important skill in sports. To achieve a firm, flat stomach, pull in your lower abs while you spin your body from side to side while engaging your abdominal muscles. The Russian twist effectively burns calories. Additionally, it strengthens the lower back and helps with balance.

How to work out:

You begin by sitting on your exercise mat with your feet flat on the floor and your knees bent.

Then, reposition yourself so that your upper body is raised 45 degrees from the ground. Throughout the workout, be sure to maintain this angle with your back straight.

Brace your core, raise your legs off the ground, and join your hands in front of your chest.

From one side to the other, fully rotate your arms.

Let's proceed to the back workout now.

SUPERMAN 10.

You must have seen Superman fly, either on a screen or in a picture, without a doubt. You're going to fly like Superman today. However, by lying on your fitness mat, you'll be able to fly. Your lower and upper back, as well as the muscles that support your spine, are strengthened by the Superman. Poor posture and discomfort can be avoided by having strong back muscles. Additionally, it tones your core, hamstrings, and glutes. Schedule the Superman in your workout if you frequently sit at a desk or experience lower back pain. This exercise is a great complement to many core workouts.

How to work out:

Start by assuming a prone position on the floor and stretching your arms and legs fully backward. You should steadily raise your arms, legs, upper back, and head off the ground while exhaling. Your hands and toes should be spaced apart from the ground, and your torso should have a small curvature. Hold this position with your body. Once you've reached your starting position, exhale.

REVERSE SNOW ANGEL, No. 11

A fantastic workout for increasing strength is the reverse snow angel. Your scapular stabilizing muscles' end ranges of control are also improved.

How to work out:

Starting position is to lay face down on your exercise mat with your arms and legs extended behind you.

Lift your arms, legs, and torso a few inches off the ground. Similar to trying to make snow angels, move your legs apart while moving your arms backward to the pelvis.

Go back to your starting point. That represents.

12. STONE ROW

Plank Row has several uses. The exercise is comprehensive because it uses your arms, legs, and abs. Plank Row strengthens your back, chest, shoulders, neck, and abs, which makes it simpler to maintain neutral posture with your shoulders back and lower back in a neutral position. Your upper body rotation is aided, and your balance is enhanced. It works your core, improves spinal stability, and strengthens your shoulder, arm, and upper back muscles. Basically, this exercise covers everything you can imagine.

How to work out:

Your legs should be hip-width apart as you begin in the plank posture. Make sure your hands are piled beneath your shoulders and that your back is straight.

Engage your glutes and contract your core. Exhale, stabilizing your chest as you lift one arm to row, and feel the shoulder blade on that side slipping toward your spine as you bend that elbow upward.

Repeat the motion on the other side after lowering the arm to the floor.

The checklist item for the back has been checked off. The chest will come next.

13. EXCEL

A common and well-liked exercise that is great for developing upper body and core strength is the push-up. It's so well-liked for a reason, and that reason is that they are incredible. It is a compound exercise that, when performed correctly, partially engages the muscles in the legs, back, triceps, chest, and shoulders. The push-up comes in countless varieties. You should begin with the leisurely versions as a beginner and work your way up to the more difficult ones as you advance.

How to work out:

Get on the ground and assume the press-up position. Your fingers should be facing forward, and your arms should be somewhat out from your shoulders. On your hands and toes, maintain equilibrium. Without arching your back or sagging in the midsection, let your body to be in a straight line from your head to your toes. Depending on what's comfortable for you, you can spread your feet apart or keep them close together.

Before beginning any movements, tighten your core and contract your abs. Throughout the entire push-up, make sure your muscles are flexed.

Inhale as you slowly lower yourself until your elbows are at a 90-degree angle.

Exhale as you begin to tighten your chest muscles and return to the starting posture by pushing through your hands.

There are numerous push-up varieties, as I've already mentioned. I'll sum up a few.

BROAD PUSH-UP

It is a good exercise for strengthening the upper body and core. Compared to a regular push-up, it concentrates more on the chest and shoulder muscles while also exercising the muscles next to the chest. While doing all of this, the muscles in the neck and back are supported. Additionally, it improves balance and posture, strengthens the core, and safeguards the back from harm.

How to work out:

Your hands should be wider than your shoulders when you begin in the plank posture. You want your fingers pointing forward.

As you drop your body toward the floor, bend your elbows out to the sides. Once your chest is below your elbows, stop.

As you press into your hands and raise your body back to the beginning position, keep your core tight.

DOUBLE PUSH-UP

It is sometimes referred to as a triangle push-up. This push-up variation is a complex workout and a step up from the basic push-up. Compared to a regular pushup, a diamond pushup concentrates more on and on your triceps. It's ideal for getting your arms ready for additional exercises like pull-ups or bench presses with a close grip. As a complex exercise, it engages shoulder muscles like the anterior deltoid and chest muscles like the pectoralis major.

Start your workout by assuming the plank posture. You can set your legs hip-width apart or together. The secret to this exercise is to form a diamond shape by joining your thumbs and index fingers. Tuck your elbows in close to your body and engage your core. Then, as you lower your torso toward your hands until your upper arms are next to your ribcage, bend your elbows. As you do this, your shoulder blades should retract. Squeeze your chest and straighten your elbows to get back to the beginning position while maintaining good technique. As you come back, your shoulder blades should retract. Squeeze your chest and triceps as you stand back up.

Incline When performing a push-up, spread your hands somewhat beyond shoulder width on a bench or box. Bend your arms and go low till your chest meets the bench or box with your feet firmly planted on the ground. Reverse the process by raising your body back to the beginning position.

Decline Push-up: Your feet should be on a bench or box, and your hands should be firmly planted on the floor. Your body should be lowered so that your chest is virtually on the floor. After a brief pause, push your body back up to the starting position and repeat. If you were a beginner, using a low box would be beneficial.

The one-arm pushup and clap pushup are only two of the several other push-up types. These, however, are extremely tough and offer minimal advantages over the earlier forms. If I'm being completely honest, I believe that these methods are frequently employed to demonstrate one's strength rather than to develop muscle. You may easily increase the number of reps or use resistance bands to provide more resistance if you find the push-ups to be too simple. Don't worry, though; we'll discuss that later.

STAR PLANK 14.

The star plank tones your complete core in addition to your obliques. Your shoulders and arms get stronger, but your hip and oblique muscles get deeply contracted. Additionally, plank postures strengthen your intellect and willpower because maintaining the position calls for some mental toughness. Additionally, it gives you a chance to practice effective breathing. Be remember to breathe deeply while performing this workout.

How to work out:

Walk your hands and feet outward from a push-up position until they resemble an x.

To maintain a level line from your head to your hips, engage your core. from your hips to your feet after that

After maintaining that posture, proceed to resume a push-up.

REACH UNDER PLANK 15.

The abs and, to a lesser extent, the lower back, obliques, and shoulders are the primary focus of plank reach.

How to work out:

Start in a plank position, place your hands under your shoulders, maintain your back straight, and engage your abs. Keep your body in plank position. Raise an arm off the floor and place a hand on the hip on the other side. Repeat on the other side, then go back to your starting position.

We now move on to the final but most definitely not least item. Let's practice our arms.

The arms have traditionally been regarded as the hardest body-weight exercises to perform effectively. in particular the biceps. People tend to forget that we can make resistance in our limbs, which is far from the fact. The fact that you may choose how much resistance you provide is the best part. Prepare yourself as we disprove all of the skeptics.

A side-lying bicep curl, or 16.

Although it may seem strange, the side-lying bicep curl is a great alternative to the bicep curl with weights. However, mastering the right form for using the movement successfully takes practice and is not simple. It exercises the brachialis and brachioradialis muscles in your lower arm as well as the biceps muscles on the front of your upper arm. You employ these muscles on a daily basis. The side-lying bicep curl exercise helps you learn how to use your arm muscles while strengthening your upper arm.

How to work out:

Lie on any side, but for the purposes of this tutorial, we'll say left. After that, squat and flex your waist.

Behind your head, place your right hand.

While flexing your torso simultaneously, grab your left leg with your left hand and pull steadily.

Then, hold the contraction for a few seconds.

Keeping hold of your leg, bring your body back down.

LEG BARBELL CURL 17.

In basic form, this biceps workout is pretty simple. But keep in mind that you can create resistance by pressing your legs up against your arms. The resistance increases as you move farther from your arms.

How to work out:

Stand against the wall to start this workout. With your palm facing up, grasp your right ankle with your left hand.

As high as you can, lift your ankle toward your shoulder, pause for a little moment, and then lower it. That represents. For the other side, repeat.

COBRA PUSH-UP 18.

A terrific bodyweight workout for the triceps is the Cobra push-up. It increases the weight loaded through the triceps while also working the hips.

How to work out:

Lie on the floor with your thighs and chest parallel to the surface. Spread your palms out so they are broader than a shoulder's breadth on the floor.

Keep the lower half against the floor and raise the upper body off of it.

Then, lower yourself back to your starting position after holding this position for 5 seconds.

Chapter 6

PERCENTAGE OF BODYWEIGHT IN TRICEPS

A calisthenics exercise known as the bodyweight triceps extension primarily targets the triceps and, to a lesser extent, the lower back and shoulders. You could do a lot of various variations. Others call for the use of a barbell and squat rack. But since that isn't the topic of this chapter, our attention will be only on your body weight.

How to work out:

Beginning with all four. Almost identical to the push-up starting position, with the exception that your hands are slightly forward of your shoulders rather than precisely beneath them. On your hands and toes, maintain equilibrium.

As opposed to a traditional push-up, you slowly lower yourself until your elbows contact the floor and your hands are in a L shape.

A rep is when you get back to your starting position.

My list of challenging bodyweight exercises comes to an end here. In order to provide you the finest bodyweight training possible and to make a point, I want to remind you of all of the stated exercises before going on to the next chapter. To put it another way, you can maintain a perfectly balanced exercise program without spending any money. The beauty of it is that. Anyone can exercise; how you exercise is entirely up to you.

CPSIA information can be obtained
at www.ICGtesting.com
Printed in the USA
LVHW040111060123
736479LV00011B/985

9 781801 899239